Preface

My hope for this diet plan is that it will help you quickly learn about healthy food choices and not only lose weigh but keep it off. I have worked for years helping others with their weight struggles but it was not until I had my first child that I truly understood how difficult it can be to lose excess weight and keep it off. The most frustrating part for me was that as a new Mom I didn't have any time. How was I suppose to fit in exercise and prepare healthy meals when I had this new bundle of joy that needed my constant attention 24 hours a day, 7 days a week. I know time is a precious commodity for most of us and it is for this reason that I developed the No Nonsense diet plan. I certainly did not have time to read a 200 page book on nutrition after my daughter was born and my guess is you don't either. My hope is that this concise and simple plan will fit your busy lifestyle and help you reach your weight loss goals.

Introduction

There is nothing magical about losing weight. However, there is a lot of misinformation about nutrition floating around due to the latest fad diets. Therefore, it is not surprising that Americans continue to gain weight despite the vast amount of money that is spent on trying to lose it! Two thirds of Americans are overweight and obesity contributes to five of the ten leading causes of death. There is no great secret that anyone can tell you that can offer a quick fix. Successful weight loss is truly basic math and comes down to the amount of calories you consume vs. the amount of calories you burn. Thus, if you decrease the amount of food you consume and increase your activity level you will lose weight. However, this is easier said than done and often people are left wondering what foods are good for them to eat and which ones are not. I truly believe that the key is MODERATION! No foods are off limit but some are obviously better choices than others. If you can balance your food choices in moderation you will have a healthy diet and lose weight. I look at weight loss as a triad or a triangle with each side representing an equal and important part of weight loss. The three sides of the triangle are: 1. Psychological/behavioral change, 2. Nutrition and 3. Exercise. Without one of the sides the triangle will fall and the same is true for weight loss. If you do not commit to working on all sides of the triad you will not be successful in losing weight. I wrote this book to give you the knowledge and tools to achieve the weight loss triad and develop a plan that you can live with for life. (Please note that you should always consult your physician before starting a new diet or exercise regimen.)

Be realistic!

Most of us live very crazy lives and the thought of adding anything else to our crazy schedules is daunting. That is why it is so important to look at losing weight as a marathon and not a sprint. As much as we would all like to be able to lose 20 pounds overnight, it is not only unrealistic but unachievable as well. A weight loss goal of one to two pounds per week is not only realistic but will provide you with results that will be long lasting. The idea of this plan is to make small changes overtime that you will stick with for life and can incorporate easily into your daily routine. This will prevent you from feeling overwhelmed and causing you to throw in the towel. Remember that you will have good days and bad days and that is to be expected. If you have a day in which you eat foods that are not the best choices, and trust me there will be days like this, there is no need to beat yourself up! Remember that losing weight and having a healthy lifestyle are about making the best choices you can most of the time but not all of the time. If you have a bad day or you overeat on a holiday, there is no need to give up but instead put it behind you and start making better choices at your next meal. This is not about being perfect but about being realistic and living a long healthy life.

Psychology of Eating

Let me be clear in stating that I am not by any means a psychiatrist, psychologist or a therapist nor would I ever claim to be. However, if you work in the nutrition/weight loss field it does not take long to realize that losing weight has a huge psychological component. In fact, often times weight issues have very little if anything to do with food. It is imperative for people who want to lose weight to first analyze how and why they became overweight in the first place. Was it simply poor food choices and lack of exercise or was it something deeper like emotional eating. Until one truly recognizes what causes him or her to be overweight he/she will never successfully lose and keep the weight off. I am not suggesting that once you have identified what type of eater you are that you need to announce your findings to a room full of strangers. This revelation is for your own growth and development only. The goal is for you to be able to identify what motivates you to overeat so that you can tailor a diet plan accordingly. It is my opinion that everyone who needs to lose weight will fit into the following three groups described in the next paragraph. Take time to thoroughly analyze which group you fall into and be honest with yourself so that you will be able to begin the journey to a healthier lifestyle.

Types of "Eaters"!

In my experience there are three types of "eaters". There are psychological eaters, behavioral eaters and eaters who are a combination of both the psychological and behavioral eater. The most important step that you can and must take in order to lose weight is to figure out what type of eater you are. Most importantly you must be honest with your self about your eating habits and be aware of what you are putting in your body.

Psychological eaters are people who eat to suppress feelings. Early on in life these types of eaters developed an unhealthy relationship with food and often use food as a coping mechanism. They may have even had a traumatic event in their life such as being physically or mentally abused as a child.

When they are sad they eat to make themselves feel better and if they are happy they eat to celebrate. When you are a true psychological eater there is no diet in the world that will completely fix your issues with food. Food is not your problem but instead a symptom of a deeper underlying issue. It is best for psychological eaters to work with a psychologist and/or counselors in addition to working on their diet in order to help address the root of what causes them to overeat.

Behavioral eaters choose what to eat out of habit and or convenience. They may indeed be clueless as to how to eat healthy. Eating for them is a learned behavior and these people have not yet learned the skills to eat a healthful diet. Often times behavioral eaters grew up in homes in which healthy choices were not a part of their normal diet. They might also eat out of boredom and or convenience using a lot of pre-packaged or fast food items. However, given the proper tools and skills these types of eaters can change their habits and lose weight successfully. You may also fit into this group if your weight gain is due to a specific event such as pregnancy or if your suffered an injury.

Finally, some people fall in the middle and display characteristics of both psychological and behavioral eaters. They will have to address issues in both categories to overcome their weight problems.

Food Journaling

I am often asked if you should write down every morsel of food that you put in your mouth when you are trying to lose weight. My feelings on this are mixed. If you have identified that you are a true emotional eater this may be beneficial for you. You may find that writing down your food choices when you are in emotional turmoil is not only cathartic but also very revealing as well. We all tend to underestimate how much we are actually consuming. Writing down the types of food and amounts can make us aware of where we need to improve our diets. I would suggest that everyone spend 3 to 5 days journaling what they are consuming. This is usually enough time to uncover a typical pattern of eating. For emotional eaters you may want to continue to journal longer if you find it beneficial. I would caution that if journaling becomes so overwhelming that it causes you to want to quit than it is time to stop. It should not become all consuming.

Food Basics

The key to a healthy diet is a balanced diet. It is beneficial to have some form of protein, carbohydrate and fat at every meal. Each brings an important element to the meal. Let's explore what each has to offer.

Carbohydrates are the major source of energy for our bodies and each gram of carbohydrate provides four calories per gram. Since glucose is the main fuel for the brain, carbohydrates are an essential part of our diet. Carbohydrates are found primarily in plant based products such as grains, fruits and vegetables. Carbohydrates can be broken down into two types, simple and complex. Simple Carbohydrates like white table sugar for example are used quickly in your body and will give you a burst of energy because they cause a spike in blood sugar. While they will give you a quick burst of energy they may also leave you feeling sluggish when the effect wears off. Complex carbohydrates like wheat bread or brown rice are processed more slowly thus, not producing as drastic of a spike in blood sugar. Because they are usually higher in fiber they give you a greater feeling of satiety.

Protein plays a crucial role in the synthesis of tissue and metabolic functions. It provides the amino acids needed to build and maintain muscle. One gram of protein provides four calories per gram and is found mostly in meat, dairy and nuts. The best lean cuts of meat for a healthy diet are those with little to no marbling (fat) and without skin. When choosing dairy look for the low fat or fat free variety.

Fat is an essential part to everyone's diet but unfortunately fat gets a bad rap. Fat helps transport fat soluble vitamins and is an essential part of cell membranes. Each fat gram contains nine calories per gram. Fat helps give food flavor and provides a high satiety (fullness) factor. There are three basic types of fat: saturated, polyunsaturated and monounsaturated.

Saturated fats are found in animal products such as dairy, beef, chicken, pork and vegetable products such as coconut and palm oil. With the exception of coconut oil, saturated fat is hard at room temperature and thus, is the fat that clogs arteries. Examples of saturated fats are butter, lard, bacon grease and meat fat (marbling).

Polyunsaturated fats are a good source of omega three and omega six fatty acids. Examples of polyunsaturated fats are corn oil, sunflower and safflower oils. Polyunsaturated fat is liquid at room temperature.

Monounsaturated fats are the least artery clogging fat. Examples of monounsaturated fat are nuts, avocados, olive, canola, and peanut oil. Monounsaturated fat is liquid at room temperature.

Trans-fatty acids are unsaturated fats that have been hydrogenated to make them semisolid and act more like saturated fat. These types of fats are found in high fat baked goods, snacks, stick margarine and commercial frying fats. It is best to limit the amount of trans fat in your diet as they act like saturated fat and can help lead to blocked arteries.

Try thinking of your arteries like pipes. If you have ever melted butter you know that at room temperature it hardens. Now visualize pouring butter down your pipes (arteries) and remember when it hardens it will coat your arteries and eventually cause build up. However, when you have a bottle of oil (mono or polyunsaturated) it is liquid at room temperature and will slide down your pipes (arteries) rather than clog and cause build up.

What are you drinking?

You would probably be very surprised to find out how many calories are in everyday beverages. It is common for many people to have two to three cans of soda a day plus a glass of juice in the morning.

One 12oz can of coca cola is 140 calories while a 12oz glass of juice can be 195calories. A couple of cans of soda and a glass of juice a day equal almost 500 calories which translates into one extra pound of fat a week! This is not to say that you can't ever have a can of soda but you need to be aware of how many calories you are downing. Choosing diet soda can be a good alternative but increasing your water consumption and drinking skim milk is your best options. When you do decide to have a glass of juice make sure that it is a 100% juice you are drinking instead of a "juice cocktail" which can contain more sugar than actual juice. Always keep in mind that most of the glasses that people have in their homes can hold at least 12oz of liquid making it very easy to down 300 calories in one large gulp. Try to fill the glass half way or look for smaller juice glasses to have your morning orange juice. You can also dilute juice with regular or sparkling water to save yourself half the calories of a full glass of juice. Remember that juice contains little to no fiber so eating the actual fruit such, as an orange will give you a greater feeling of fullness.

When should I eat?

Clients often ask me if they can skip meals like breakfast or lunch in favor of having a larger meal at dinner time. My answer to this is always a firm no! In theory, if a person is on an 1800 calorie diet and sticks firm to this diet; it should not matter if the person has three meals, six meals or one meal to achieve this amount of calories per day. However, studies show that for people who wait to eat all day for a big meal at night are so famished that they tend to overeat by 400 to 600 calories therefore, sabotaging their diet plan. It is always better to fuel your body throughout the day to keep you satisfied enough to not overeat and most importantly make healthy choices. Most people can relate to having a day in which they did not eat breakfast and lunch only to come home and raid the kitchen cabinets for anything to satisfy their hunger. By fueling throughout the day your chances of this happening decrease significantly. Eating throughout the day gives your body the chance of burning off some calories during the day instead of just going to bed after a large dinner.

Be present when you eat!

One of the worst diet sabotages is the television. We
live is such a face paced world that it is so tempting
to come home grab a snack and sit on the coach
eating while we watch a show. The problem is that
most people are so tuned-in to what they are
watching that before they know it they have
devoured an entire bag of some sort of snack food
without realizing it. The same is true if you find
yourself eating more than one meal a day on the run
in your car. When you are trying to stick to a
healthy diet, it is best to try to have as many meals
as you can at a table without the television on. This
way you can enjoy your meal without distraction
and be aware of what you are putting in your
mouth. In most areas of our lives we value
presentation and why should meal times at home be
any different. By setting the table and lighting a few
candles, it just may relax you enough to slow down,
savor and enjoy a meal.

Slow it down!

I think we all can admit to rolling ourselves away from the table when we have had too much to eat. You may wonder how it is that one minute you can be happily eating turkey at Thanksgiving and the next minute feel as though you are beyond stuffed. Unfortunately, it can take your stomach up to twenty minutes to sense and tell your brain to stop eating because you are full. For this very reason many of us overeat. If this is something you feel that you fall victim to, the only way to overcome this is to slow it down. Take your time eating your meal and when you have finished a serving wait at least twenty minutes before having another. You may find that after the time has passed that you are no longer hungry. The natural hunger cues that we were born with that tell us when we are hungry and when we are full, are often "confused" by the time we reach adult hood. If you were a child who grew up in a family that made you finish your plate before leaving the table, you probably are no longer in tune with your natural hunger cues. When we are children our bodies tell us when we have had enough, but if your parents forced you to clean your plate you may have learned to ignore you body's natural response to fullness in order to obey your parents. By slowing down your eating and waiting between courses you can learn to listen to your body and your natural hunger cues.

Food Group Basics

Let us review the basics of the food groups and which food choices are the best from each group.

Fruits and Vegetable: Everything in this group is pretty much a go! A good rule of thumb when choosing vegetables is the brighter the color the more nutrients the vegetable contains. For example: iceberg lettuce is very low in any nutrients at all and is mostly water. However, romaine lettuce or any dark green lettuce is packed with vitamins and antioxidants making them much better choices than the old stand by of iceberg. While fresh vegetables are usually considered the best, frozen and some canned vegetables can be great choices as well. In fact nutrients can be lost in fresh vegetables due to the fact that they are picked weeks before they reach their final destination. During this time of exposure to light, shipping and storage many vitamins and minerals are lost. With canned and frozen vegetables they are usually processed within days of being harvested and thus, more of the vitamins and minerals are preserved. While it is true that these nutrients can be lost during processing, it is usually no more than is lost in fresh fruits and veggies during transit. The one area of caution with canned vegetables is the high amounts of sodium. This can easily be avoided by buying low salt versions of your favorite canned veggies.

Fresh fruit is always an integral part of a healthy diet plan. If your favorite fruit is not in season, frozen or canned fruit can be a great and affordable alternative. When choosing canned fruit try to buy fruit in light syrup or fruit in its natural juices rather than fruit in heavy syrup; this will save you a lot of extra calories.

Cooking Methods: The best way to prepare your veggies is to bake, steam or grill rather than boiling.

These choices are better than boiling because when you boil vegetables you may end up destroying many of the nutrients by the high temperatures. When you drain boiled veggies you are pouring off all of the vitamins and minerals that you have boiled right out of your vegetable. Steaming, baking or grilling will help preserve those vitamins and minerals. It is easier now more than ever to steam or bake vegetables. Many frozen veggies now come in microwave safe bags that can be taken out of the freezer and put directly into your microwave and cooked within minutes. When using fresh veggies you can easily dice them and place them on a cookie sheet with non stick spray or a little olive oil to bake. You can also put sliced fresh veggies in a microwavable dish and steam until tender. Both methods are easy and preserve the vitamins and minerals in the veggies.

Dairy Group: I am a huge fan of the dairy group because it is the best way for you to get the much needed calcium and vitamin D that your body needs. The key is to choose low fat dairy that is high in calcium and vitamin D but low in the saturated fat that can clog your arteries. You don't have to go as far as fat free dairy products but low fat varieties are very good and save you a lot of calories and fat. Often times you can't really tell the difference between low fat cheese and yogurt from the full fat variety. When choosing milk, skim would be optimal but I fully realize that a comment like this could cause many of you reading this to throw this book out the window! Skim may be too extreme, so the best idea is to try the next lower fat variety of the milk that you are drinking now. For example if you are drinking whole milk, try 2%, if you are drinking 2% try 1% and so on. After a couple of months on the lower fat variety, challenge yourself to try the next lower fat version until you ultimately end with 1% or skim. There are some great companies that make lower fat milks like Smart Milk that are creamier than other low fat varieties. These companies use milk solids to thicken the milk so that it feels thicker and creamier but is still low in fat. I strongly encourage you to try these. This type of product may be just the key to tricking yourself into drinking lower fat milk.

Meat group: It is so easy now to find lean cuts of meat in the grocery store. Chicken not only comes skinless and boneless but also in individual packets to make it super easy to make a few servings at a time and freeze the rest. Ground chicken and turkey are readily available in local grocery stores as well. Little packets of chicken tenderloins take no more than 15 min in the oven, and you have a healthy low fat protein for lunch or dinner. The key with choosing a low fat protein is to look for meats that are skinless and have very little visible fat or marbling like pork tenderloin or filet mignon. If you find yourself with a package of pork chops or beef that is fattier than you would like, simply trim all visible fat before cooking. Ground meat can be a great option for dinner as well, just look for very lean varieties like ground white meat chicken, turkey or 96% lean ground beef. These can be used to make all of the favorite dishes you grew up with like meatballs, chili and meatloaf. Fish and shellfish are great lean protein sources and take minutes to cook. Even high fat fish like Salmon are great choices because they are rich in heart healthy fats like omega 3 fatty acid. The same is true for eggs. It is fine to have a few eggs a week in moderation or if you enjoy them daily alternate between whole eggs and using egg whites. You can purchase egg whites in a carton that are a great low fat substitute for eggs. They can be used for cooking or baking.

Cooking methods: The best way to reduce fat when cooking meat is to stick to grilling, baking, or boiling meat. These methods require little if any extra fat to be added to the meat when cooking. Frying or sautéing adds extra fat to the meat you are preparing therefore, increasing the amount of calories in the meal.

Bread and Starch group: The bottom line with this group is fiber! When we talk about complex and simple forms of carbohydrates, it is really referring to the amount of fiber in these types of foods. When choosing bread products, pasta or rice you want to look for whole wheat varieties. The whole wheat varieties are less processed than the white and take longer to break down once eaten. Thus, the same amount of whole wheat pasta will make you feel more full than the same amount of white pasta.

Manufactures of food products have really met the demand of consumers by increasing the number of products on the market that are of the whole wheat variety. You can find whole wheat bread, waffles, hamburger buns and pasta. It is easy to integrate these whole wheat varieties into your diet. My suggestion would be to try a couple of new whole wheat varieties a week until you can slowly phase out as many of the white varieties in your diet as possible. Be flexible and willing to try different brands. Just like white bread not every manufacturer of wheat bread makes a good product therefore; be patient and willing to try a few different brands until you find one that you like.

Oh the Magic of Fiber

Fiber plays a monumental role in losing weight. Fiber is found in grains, fruits and vegetables and what most people do not realize is that the more fiber you eat the fuller you feel (satiety factor). There are two types of fiber: soluble fiber and insoluble fiber; both types are an important part of a healthy diet. Soluble fiber is found in carrots, citrus fruits, apples, oats, legumes and barley. Insoluble fiber is found in whole-wheat, bran, vegetables and fruits with edible seeds. A good rule of thumb is to limit the white forms of carbohydrates in your diet and instead look for the whole wheat (brown) versions of carbohydrates. For instance white bread, pasta and rice are processed to the point where most of the fiber is removed. Thus, when it is absorbed in your body it is processed quickly like simple sugar. Whole wheat varieties are less processed and still contain the fiber that makes you feel full. For example a piece of wheat bread is a complex carbohydrate instead of a simple sugar. It is broken down more slowly in the body and does not cause a rapid spike in insulin, as white bread would. Whenever possible look for the whole wheat versions of your favorite foods such as: whole wheat bread, whole wheat English muffins, whole wheat pasta and brown rice. When you look at the food label of these foods they should have at least 2g or more of fiber per serving. I will caution you to be careful of labels such as split top or buttered wheat. Once you read the label you will realize that it is not true whole wheat bread but instead brown colored white bread.

FAB FATS!

Fat in food has been given such a bad rap in recent years that some people have become fat phobic. It truly does your diet plan an injustice to think that you should omit fat from your diet. Fat is an essential part of a healthy diet and is the main reason why we feel full and satisfied after consuming a meal. There are many different types of fat and some choices are more beneficial to your health than others. However, with that being said there does need to be a limit on how much fat you consume. Trust me, if you eat too much EVOO (extra virgin olive oil) you will end up with OBFA (one big fat, well you know what I mean)! Keep in mind that all fats have a lot of calories and a small amount goes a long way. Let us discuss the different types and which ones are most beneficial to your health.

Monounsaturated Fat: These are the best fats that you can eat. I like to think of them as the king of the castle fats. Olive, peanut and canola oil are examples of monounsaturated fat. The chemical make of this type of fat is such that it has only one double bond thus, making it easier to break down that saturated fat. These fats are not damaged by oxidation therefore; they are less likely to increase cholesterol buildup in your arteries. Again, think of your arteries like pipes and the oil easily sliding down them.

Polyunsaturated Fat: This fat is liquid at room temperature as well but instead of having one double bond like monounsaturated fat, polyunsaturated fat has two or more double bonds. Examples of polyunsaturated fats are vegetable, corn, safflower, soybean and sunflower oils. The two main types of essential polyunsaturated fats are Omega 6 linoleic and Omega 3 linolenic acid. These are essential fatty acids because our bodies can not manufacture these fats and we are dependent on food to obtain them. There have been many studies that have linked these fats with disease prevention and early brain development. These fats are better choices over saturated fat in your diet because they too are liquid at room temperature and will easily slide down your pipes!

Saturated Fat: This type of fat can cause the most harm in your diet because it is solid at room temperature and has the ability to clog your arteries. These fats are not sliding down your pipes but instead clogging up the precious space in which your blood needs to travel. Examples of saturated fat would be any animal fat like butter, marbling on meat and coconut or palm tree oils.

Trans Fat: Trans fat is manufactured fat. Manufacturers add hydrogen to liquid oil to make them semisolid at room temperature. Examples would be stick margarine, shortening, and often restaurant fried food. You will also find trans fat in a lot of packaged high-fat baked goods and snacks. Studies suggest that this type of fat can increase blood cholesterol and contribute to atherosclerosis.

The bottom line is that you need to watch the amount of calories you consume from fat, however; the calories that you do consume from fat should come from monounsaturated or polyunsaturated fat.

The skinny on low-fat products

The problem with low fat foods is not with the products themselves but the fact that people tend to feel like it is a free pass to eat as much of a particular food as they want. The truth is that even though a food may be low in fat does not mean that it is calorie free. In fact, a lot of low fat foods are filled with extra sugar to make up for the taste they lose when the fat is removed. The truth is that there are a lot of really great low fat products out there but probably just as many that are not worth your time. You need to be choosy and decide which ones you are really ready to substitute for the real thing on a daily basis. For example I really like low fat sour cream and feel that the taste difference is so minimal that I can live with this substitution. However, it does not mean that I can put a cup of sour cream on my baked potato. If you find that you consistently have to use more of a low fat product than you would of the full fat version, than you may be better off sticking to a smaller portion of the full fat version. I also find that many of the fat free versions of food are in one word un-edible like, fat free mayo. Keep in mind that with the fat removed many of these products will not fill you up and satisfy your hunger as the full fat versions will. I encourage you to try and experiment with all different brands of low fat and fat free products. You may be pleasantly surprised to find ones that you like and will save you a lot of fat and calories.

Understanding the Food Label

While food labels may look intimidating they really are easy to decipher as long as you know what you are looking for. The most important information on the food label is the serving size. First you must look at what constitutes a serving size and how many servings are in the package of food that you want to consume. For instance if you are going to eat a package of crackers and the serving size is five crackers but there are two servings per package, then you would have to multiply all the nutritional information by two. This is to account for multiple servings.

After you have established what the serving size of a particular food is then you can look at the calories, fat, carbohydrates, fiber and protein per serving depending on what is important to your diet plan. You can use this information to decide where the particular food that you want to eat fits sensibly into your diet plan.

There is no reason to look at the % of daily value for each nutrient. These values are based on a 2,000 calorie diet plan and that may or may not apply to you. It is better to stick to the actual amounts.

You will also want to look at the ingredient portion of the food label. This is where you can find out if a particular food is made of whole wheat flour or enriched wheat flour. Whenever possible choose products that are made with whole wheat flour as they are less processed and contain more fiber.

Remember the more fiber in a food the fuller you feel after you eat it.

Calories: If you are trying to lose weight this is obviously the most important number to look at. Again make sure you are taking into consideration the serving size of the portion of food that you are eating. Very rarely does the food label pertain to the whole package. It usually refers to a serving in which there are multiple servings in the package.

Fat: It is important to look at fat because even if your ultimate goal is to lose weight you want to make sure that you are losing weight with healthy food choices. This is where you can find if a particular food is high in saturated fat and or contains trans fat. The goal is to have most of the fat calories come form unsaturated fat sources.

Carbohydrates: This refers to the total amount of sugar in the food. Unless you have diabetes and are counting carbohydrates it is not imperative that you look at this number. The main concern with carbohydrates is that you are eating high quality complex carbohydrates at most meals, not necessarily the number of grams that you are consuming.

Fiber: A high fiber food is considered a food that has 5 or more grams of fiber per serving, the more fiber that you can incorporate into your diet the better. The recommended daily allowance of dietary fiber for woman is 21-25 grams and 30-38 grams per day for men.

Protein: Unless you are a vegetarian you probably do not need to be concerned with the total number of grams of protein that you are consuming in a day. Most of us who consume meat easily reach our protein needs. However, if you are concerned you can easily calculate how much protein you are getting a day by checking this part of the food label.

To weigh or not to weigh that is the question?

Don't panic I am not talking about weighing yourself on a scale! I am referring to weighing your food to make sure you have the correct portion sizes. I think we can all agree that measuring all your food all the time is not only time consuming but completely unrealistic. However, most of us underestimate how many calories we eat because we underestimate the amount or portions of the food we consume. Living in the hectic real world that we all do, no one has time to measure out all their food. What I suggest doing is to buy a very inexpensive food scale and measure out some of your favorite meals that eat you eat on a regular basis once. This will allow you to have a better idea of just how much you are eating and allow you to estimate in the future a proper portion size. For example what does 3oz of lunch meat look like? If you put a few slices of lunch meat on the scale you can quickly find out how many pieces equal 3oz (usually 3 thin slice pieces). Do you then have to measure every time you have a sandwich? NO! The idea is to do it once so that you can eyeball the amount in the future. When measuring dry goods like cereal use a bowl that you can mark with the appropriate portion size; therefore, you can quickly dole out the proper amount at each meal. This same principle can be applied to liquids. When measuring liquids you will find that most glasses are 12-16oz thus, it is very easy to drink a lot of calories in one shot. Most serving sizes of liquids are in one cup or 8oz increments and if you measure out 8oz you will probably find that it is a lot less than what most of us drink. All this measuring might lead you to the conclusion that your new food portions look too small in your bowls, glasses or plates. We live in the "Super Size it" age and our plates, glasses and utensils are no exception. Research has shown that by using smaller utensils, bowls, plates and glasses that you can actually trick yourself into eating fewer calories. If nothing else this just might be a great excuse to go out and buy some new stylish plates.

Willpower, is there such a thing?

The most difficult challenge that my clients face is avoiding any junk food that is in their houses. To be honest who could refuse chocolate, chips and cake if they were readily accessible in your kitchen cabinet. My suggestion to everyone trying to improve their diet and lose weight is to rid their house of any temptation with the exception of a few treats for special occasions. My clients usually flinch at this suggestion because these types of foods are usually in their homes because of a significant other and/ or children. "But my kids eat it", is the most common response I elicit when I dare suggest to rid your cabinets of junk. If you are trying to revamp your eating habits to lose weight and have a healthier lifestyle, doesn't it seem reasonable that if you are feeding your kids the types of foods that caused you to be in this predicament, that they too will be facing the same types of issues when they get older? Why not teach them how to enjoy healthy foods from and early age and prevent them from having weight and health issues later in life. However, significant others may pose more of a challenge but explaining to them how important it is to you to have their support can make all the difference. Most will choose to help you live a healthier life. Who knows, they may decide to join you in your quest for a more healthful lifestyle and it may be a great bonding opportunity for your entire family.

Recipe Modification

Everyone has their favorite meals or dishes that have been passed down from generation to generation. However, sometimes the foods that we grow up on are not the healthiest for us. Does that mean that we totally have to abandon our favorite dishes? The answer is a resounding no and you have two options when it comes to such meals. You can modify them to make healthier versions that more appropriately fit into your healthy diet plan. You may also choose not to change them and just have them less often on special occasions. It is very easy to make small changes to your favorite recipes to make them healthier. My suggestion is that you only make a few changes per recipe rather than making the entire recipe low fat to help preserve the integrity of the original recipe. The following chart lists the healthy substitutions you can make to improve your favorite recipes.

Traditional food	Substitution
Whole milk	Low fat milk 2%, 1% or skim
Butter	Low fat margarine
Cream	Evaporated milk
Egg	2 egg whites or 1/4 cup of egg substitute
Yogurt	Low fat or fat free yogurt
Cottage cheese	1% or fat free cottage cheese
Ricotta	Low fat or skim ricotta
1 cup shortening	2/3 cup vegetable oil
Cheese	Low fat 2%, 1% or fat free
Regular Mayo	Light mayo
Salad dressing	Low fat or fat free dressing
White flour	Substitute whole wheat flour up to half of white minus 1 Tbsp
White bread	Wheat bread
Regular Bread crumbs	Whole wheat bread crumbs
Canned fruits and veggies	Canned fruits/veggies in natural juices
Tuna fish in oil	Albacore tuna in water
Whipped cream	Low fat whipped topping
Sugar	Reduce by ¼ in baked goods
1 ounce bakers chocolate	3 Tbsp of cocoa powder and 1 Tbsp of vegetable oil

The organic debate!

I am often asked if I think it is beneficial to buy organic foods over regular food. To answer this we first need to define organic. As of October 2002, the United States Department of Agriculture (USDA) allows food manufacturers to use a seal for foods that are 95% organic. "Any remaining product ingredients must consist of nonagricultural substances approved on the National List or non-organically produced agricultural products that are not commercially available in organic food". Products that meet the standard for 100% organic may display this on their principal display panel. If a food is a 100% organic it cannot be produced using excluded methods such as sewage sludge, or ionizing radiation. If a food has at least 70% organic ingredients it can use the phrase "made with organic ingredients" on the principal display panel. The theory behind organic foods is that because they are usually grown with lower levels of pesticides they may be healthier for us. However, at this time no scientific evidence shows that these foods are healthier or safer than conventionally grown foods.

One major obstacle to consumers buying all organic food is that it can be quite pricey. My personal belief is that if affordable buying organic food is the best option. Most of us would agree that we are in favor of reducing the amount of chemicals we consume. However, if buying organic fruits and vegetables is out of your price range and would cause you to buy less of them than I would forgo organic and reap the benefit of more fruits and vegetables in your diet regardless if they are organic or not. You can use a veggie/fruit spray, that you can buy at your local super market, to spray on your non-organic produce to clean away pesticide residue. It is simple to make your own veggies spray as well with 1 cup of white vinegar, 1 cup of water, 1 Tbsp of baking soda and 20 drops of grapefruit seed extract. Combine all ingredients and store in a plastic spray bottle.

You can also save money by purchasing non organic fruits and vegetables that have a thick skin that is going to be discarded such as bananas or cantaloupe. Instead opt to use your money on organic fruits and vegetable that you eat the skins such as peaches, apples strawberries etc… Another cost saving tip is to buy fruits and vegetables that are in season and to seek out local farmers markets that often have organic locally grown food that is more cost effective than the supermarket. If you have the space, try growing your own garden for truly organic fruits and veggies that will cost you pennies.

Restaurant eating

Clients typically do not have a problem with sticking to a healthy diet at home but tend to completely panic when they are faced with restaurant dinning. While eating out does pose some issues in the sense that you are not in control of how the food is prepared, you can still find healthier options by following the guidelines in this plan. Since you will be estimating portion sizes, you will want to follow the plate diagram as a guide. For example most of your plate should be filled with high fiber veggies that are steamed, grilled or a side salad. One quarter of your plate should be a lean meat like chicken, fish, pork or lean red meat like filet mignon. Ask for the meat/fish to be baked, broiled or grilled rather than fried or sautéed which uses more fat while preparing the meat. The last quarter of your plate should be a high fiber carbohydrate like a baked potato, winter squash or corn. If you follow the plate diagram and what you have learned about healthier options in this plan you will be able to stick to these choices while dinning out. Always allow room in your diet plan for special occasions when you go all out and have the fettuccini alfredo and cheesecake for dessert!

You MUST move to LOSE!

In order for anyone to lose weight and keep weight off you MUST incorporate an exercise regime into your life. If you do not, I will guarantee that it will take you longer to lose weight and your chances of keeping it off will greatly be reduced. In order for this plan to work best you need to combine your diet with an exercise routine that you do three to five times a week. If you are currently not exercising you can start with a plan of working out three times a week for a month until you can increase your exercise level up to four or five times a week. Everyone is busy and trying to find time to exercise can seem more difficult than taking a flight to the moon; therefore, my suggestion is to first start exercising on the weekends. If you can workout on Saturday and Sunday when you are not rushing home from work then you only have to fit in one more day during the week to achieve a three day a week exercise plan. When you do exercise aim for 30 minutes of aerobic exercise followed by weight training. You by no means need to join a gym to accomplish this. You can walk or run outside or on a treadmill, or chose from thousands of work out DVD's. You can purchase inexpensive weights or resistance bands at a department store for strength training. If you do chose to go to a gym you have many different options for aerobic exercise machines or classes to keep you from getting bored. Not all gyms are expensive and you can reduce the cost by asking about family or senior discounts or by joining a local YMCA's in your community. Most insurance plans will even reimburse you a portion of your gym costs each year! At a gym you may also have the opportunity to work with an exercise physiologist who can help you create a work out plan tailored for you. Please note that exercise physiologist's are not trainers but instead board certified experts with a degree in exercise science and adhere to a strict code of ethics when working with clients. Working with weights can be dangerous if you are not properly taught how to use them. By working with an exercise physiologist you can feel an extra level of assurance that the person training you has been properly trained and did not receive a certificate off the internet. If you have any injuries that have kept you from exercising in the past you can also make an appointment with a physical therapist to learn what exercises you can do safely without further aggravating your condition. Always make sure before you begin any exercise plan to make an appointment with your physician to make sure you are able to begin exercising safely.

Make it Easy!

There are so many great convenience foods found in regular grocery stores that it would be crazy not to take advantage of these, especially because they can make our lives so much easier! Check out the produce aisles for pre cut veggies, lettuce in a bag and diced fruit. Such conveniences allow you to make a salad or a healthy snack in minutes. You can also find prepackaged snack packs of fruit and veggies that make packing a lunch a snap. If such pre-cut conveniences become to pricey the frozen food section has a large selection of precut and ready to use fruits and veggies that are usually more cost effective. Pre-sliced frozen fruit and veggies can be quickly added to any recipe for a healthy meal in minutes. Some food companies are even putting veggies in packages that can be put in a microwave and steamed right in their own packaging.

We can all agree that there are going to be days in which coming home and preparing a meal is just not feasible. Be prepared for these days with healthy frozen meals that you can keep in your freezer and heat in minutes. While I wouldn't advocate eating Lean Cuisines for dinner every night due to the high sodium content, they are certainly a great choice occasionally when you are pressed for time. Lean Cuisines are definitely a better choice than running through the McDonald's drive through! So I encourage you to take advantage of these convenience products that will make your life easier. Just make sure you read labels and follow the healthy guidelines outlined in this plan when making your choices.

It is a good idea to scout out local restaurants that offer healthy meal choices that you can grab for takeout when you are rushed. Restaurants like subway are more than happy to provide you with the nutritional breakdown of their meals so that you can make sensible choices when ordering out. Many chain restaurants will have the nutritional breakdown of their meals on line as well. Having "go to" healthy meal places like this when you are busy will help prevent the fast food drive through dinner.

To increase your veggie and fruit consumption per day leave pre cut veggies in your fridge for easy snacking. Prepackaged fruit cups, carrots with low fat dip and celery with peanut butter are easy snacks to throw in your lunch box for the day or leave them in your desk at work for a quick snack. Leaving a bowl of fruit on your table is a great way to remind you to take an apple or pear to work or school everyday. The easier you make it to reach for healthy alternatives the more apt you are to eat them!

Calcium

There has been some very promising research linking increase calcium intake with weight lose. Research has shown that when people have a 1,000 to 1,200 mg per day intake of calcium they lose two times the amount of fat than research participants who did not consume a high calcium diet. Increase calcium intake has also been linked to decrease cholesterol levels and osteoporosis. I strongly encourage you to drink 2 to 3 (8oz) glasses of skim milk each day in addition to other low fat dairy products. As long as you are choosing low fat versions of dairy products they will benefit your overall diet plan.

Calories: How many is too many?

In theory it is very easy to calculate how many calories you require in a day. Once you calculate your caloric needs you can simply subtract five hundred for a loss of 1 pound per week. The issue is that for most people trying to lose weight, they are already consuming more calories than they technically require and if they are put on a low calorie diet they will be hungry and unsatisfied. This is the reason why so many people abandon their weight loss program. To avoid this pitfall it is best to start with a moderate calorie diet and slowly reduce your intake. First, focus on incorporating healthy food choices into your diet and then reduce your calorie intake to a comfortable amount. Keep in mind that it can take up to twenty minutes for your stomach to tell your brain that you're full. If you feel unsatisfied at the end of a meal and want to reach for seconds, do so in this order: first, have more non-starchy vegetables, second, have more protein and third, have more whole grain carbohydrate. If you are adamant on having a number amount of calories you should eat daily as a starting point go to www.mypyramid.gov and select the tab "My Pyramid Plan". You will be asked to input your age, sex, weight, height and physical activity, the computer will then accurately calculate your calorie requirements for weight loss (this is a free service provided by the government). It is important to note that you never want to consume less than 1200 calories a day as this will slow your metabolism. Keep in mind that a healthy weight loss plan is one in which you lose 1-2 pounds per week; remember this is a marathon not a sprint!

Jacqui's Top 5 Diet Plan Offenders!

1. Soda
2. Juice (including Gatorade, Vitamin water etc…)
3. Fast Food
4. Alcohol
5. Inactivity

Maintenance: Plate Diagram

The goal of this plan is first to teach you the basics of good nutrition, second to provide you with a sample diet plan as a guide to what a healthy meal plan and proper portion control look like and third to provide you with a plan to continue with healthy eating habits for the rest of your life. The third piece of this plan is the plate diagram (please see page 67). The plate diagram is divided into three sections. First the plate is divided in half; this one half is to be filled with non-starchy vegetables. The second half of the plate is divided into half again with one section to be filled with lean protein and the other with high fiber carbohydrates (starch). The goal is to follow this plate diagram at most meal times, usually lunch and dinner as it may be more difficult to incorporate veggies into your breakfast meal. At breakfast you can substitute a serving of fruit for the veggies. The sample meal plan contained in this book is based on this plate diagram. After you feel that you have mastered portion sizes the plate diagram is an easy way to follow a healthy diet rather than measuring out all your food or obsessing about counting calories. You can follow this plan whether you are at home or at a restaurant.

You have already learned about lean protein and high fiber carbohydrates, but what are non starchy vegetables? Non starchy vegetables are vegetables that are high in fiber but very low in calories. They provide you with vitamins, minerals and fiber to fill you up with out adding extra calories. Most vegetables fit this category with the exception of a few that must be considered part of the carbohydrate category rather than the vegetable category. These vegetables are potatoes, beans, winter squash, corn and peas. Such veggies are to be counted as the carbohydrate quarter of the plate rather than the vegetable side. While it is important to have the proper portion of protein and carbohydrate at meal times, the amount of non starchy vegetable you consume should be unlimited. These vegetables are good for you and so low in calories that I do not put a limit on how much you can have at meals. Plus, very few people will overdose on broccoli!

Diet Plan

The following diet plan is meant to be a guide for what a healthy meal plan and portion control looks like. To use the plan effectively you are to choose one selection from the breakfast, lunch and dinner choices each day and add one to three snacks per day based on your caloric needs. Please note that the calorie amounts are approximate and not exact as they may differ slightly depending on which brands of food you purchase. Lower carbohydrate substitutions will have an * for people with diabetes who would like a lower carbohydrate option. Please note that carbohydrate amounts have been adjusted (fiber deducted from total carbohydrate amount) for foods containing greater than 5g of fiber per serving. Beverages are not included in the plan and my suggestion is that you have water or non-caloric drinks with your meals. Non-fat milk is a great addition to a meal as well, be sure to count the calories from the milk into your plan, one 8oz glass of skim milk is 90 calories. You may not like every meal option so feel free to pick and choose as you like however, the goal is not to eat the same foods every day. A well balanced diet is one in which there is variety; therefore, it is important to incorporate different foods that contain an array of vitamins, minerals and antioxidants in your diet. The idea of this plan is to give you the feel of what your plate should look like at meal times not to have you follow this specific diet forever. Once you feel that you understand healthy meal planning and portion control I encourage you to switch to the plate diagram and start incorporating other food options and healthy favorites into your diet.

Breakfast

- Whole wheat Lenders bagel with 2 Tbsp of light garden vegetable or plain cream cheese. (~240 calories, 57 grams of carbohydrate)

- Thomas Hearty Grain English muffin 100% whole wheat with 2 Tbsp of natural creamy peanut butter and 1 clementine. (~364 calories, 38 grams of carbohydrate)

- Two whole wheat Nutrigrain waffles with 1/4 cup of maple syrup, 1 Tbsp of Brumble and Brown butte and ½ cup of blueberries. (~485 calories, 97 grams of carbohydrate)

  *Substitute ¼ cup of Vermont sugar free syrup for the maple syrup. Total calories 290, 47 grams of carbohydrate

- 1 Packet of organic instant oatmeal made with water. Enjoy with ½ cup of 1% cottage cheese and 8 strawberries. (~300 calories, 43 grams of carbohydrate)

- Home made egg sandwich: whole wheat English muffin toasted ¼ cup egg beaters and 1 slice of American cheese. While toasting English muffin, microwave ¼ cup of egg beaters in a microwave safe bowl for 1 minute or until cooked. Then melt 1 slice of cheese on egg approximately 10 sec more in microwave. Place on English muffin. Have sandwich with a small pear. (~316 calories, 45 grams of carbohydrate)

- 1 ½ cup of Raisin Bran with ¾ cup of skim milk and a clementine (~386 calories, 75 grams of carbohydrate)

- 1 ½ cups of Cheerios with ¾ cup of skim milk and 1 cup of cut cantaloupe topped with ¼ cup pf 1% cottage cheese. (~322 calories, 61 grams of carbohydrate)

- 2 eggs (scrambled or fried with Pam), 2 slices of light wheat bread with 1 Tbsp of Brumble and

Brown margarine and 1 cup of strawberries
(about 8). (~365 calories, 35 grams of
carbohydrate)

- Chobani Greek yogurt (vanilla nonfat) with 3
  Tbsp of Cascadian Farms Granola (oats and
  honey flavor) and 1 cup of mixed berries. (~280
  calories, 47 grams of carbohydrate)

- French toast:
  2 Slices of light whole wheat bread dipped in ¼
  cup of egg beaters. Cook in a fry pan   with
  Pam. Enjoy with 1 Tbsp of Brumble and Brown
  margarine, ¼ cup maple syrup and an apple.
  (~525 calories, 86 grams of carbohydrate)

  *Substitute ¼ cup of Vermont sugar free syrup
  for ¼ cup of maple syrup = 325 calories, 41
  grams of carbohydrate.

Lunch

Free Salad: Any combination of dark greens such as romaine, spinach, bib or spring mix lettuce with peppers, tomatoes, seedless cucumbers (with skin), carrots, onions, radices. Flat out roll ups can be found in the deli section of your local grocery store, if you can't find them you can substitute another brand with approximately 100 calories per wrap.

- Multi Grain Flat Out roll up with 4oz of lean turkey breast and 1 slice of American cheese and mustard. Have with a free salad and 2 Tbsp of light salad dressing. (~380 calories, 25 grams of carbohydrate)

- Whole wheat hamburger bun with a Garden burger, topped with any of the following mustard, ketchup, lettuce, tomato and onion. Have with ½ cup of baby carrots and 1oz of baked potato chips. (~370calories, 65 grams of carbohydrate)

- Joseph's 100% flax oat bran whole wheat pita regular size with 3oz of white albacore tuna in water mixed with 2 Tbsp of light mayo, top with lettuce, tomato and onion. Have with a pear. (~400 calories, 25 grams of carbohydrate)

- Wheat Flat Out Roll up with 4oz of lean ham and 1 slice of Swiss cheese with mustard. Have with 1oz of baked chips. (~430 calories, 45 grams of carbohydrate)

- Two slices of light whole wheat bread with 4oz of lean roast beef and one slice of American cheese with 1 Tbsp of horseradish sauce or light mayo. Have with 3oz of baby carrots. (~405 calories, 31grams of carbohydrate)

- Free salad topped with 1 oz of gorgonzola cheese and 4 oz of grilled chicken breast with 2 Tbsp of light salad dressing. Have with a whole wheat pita pocket. (~358 calories, 13 grams of carbohydrate

- Free salad topped with ¼ cup of chick peas and 3oz of white tuna. Top with light salad dressing or 2 tsp of extra virgin olive oil and unlimited vinegar. Have with a whole wheat pita pocket. (~375 calories, 23 grams of carbohydrate)

- 4oz of extra lean sirloin (96/4) ground beef hamburger topped with tomato, lettuce and onion on a whole wheat bun. Enjoy with 3oz of baby carrots and 1 oz of baked potato chips. (~400 calories, 50 grams of carbohydrate)

- 4oz of flank steak grilled or broiled with Montreal Steak seasoning served on top of a free salad with 2 Tbsp of light dressing (any variety). Enjoy with a whole wheat roll. (~472 calories, 35 grams of carbohydrate)

- Chicken sausage (any flavor such as garlic, sun dried tomato etc…) grilled on a whole wheat hot dog roll. Top with unlimited grilled peppers and onions. Enjoy with 1 oz of baked chips and a Clementine. (~ 445 calories, 50 grams of carbohydrate)

Dinner

- Rosemary pork tenderloin, green beans and sweet potato dinner

-Rub 1 pound pork tenderloin with 1 tsp of extra virgin olive oil (EVOO), season with fresh or dried rosemary, Montréal steak seasoning, salt and pepper. Bake at 400 degrees until meat thermometer reaches 170 degrees. Have a 6oz serving (1 pound pork tenderloin makes approximately two and a half 6oz servings)
-Baked sweet potato with 1 Tbsp of Brumble and Brown margarine
- Roast an unlimited amount of green beans tossed with 1 Tsp of EVOO at 400 degrees for 12-15 minutes.
(~477 calories, 30 grams of carbohydrate)

- Onion pork tenderloin, zucchini and brown rice dinner

-Rub 1 pound of pork tenderloin with 1 tsp of EVOO and season with salt and pepper. Top with 2 sliced onions. Bake at 400 degrees until meat thermometer reaches 170 degrees. Have a 6oz serving.
-Slice up 2 zucchini's and 1 summer squash and toss with 1 tsp of EVOO, salt and pepper. Roast at 400 degrees for 15 minutes or until soft, makes two servings.
-Serve with 1/2 cup of brown rice
(~408 calories, 35 grams of carbohydrate)

- Tilapia (or other white fish i.e. cod, haddock) and asparagus dinner

-Mix a 1/8 cup of whole wheat bread crumbs with 1 Tbsp of melted Brumble and Brown margarine. Top a 6 oz Tilapia filet and bake at 400 degrees until cooked through and flaky.

-Unlimited asparagus, roast asparagus with 1 tsp of EVOO at 400 degrees for 12-15 minutes or until desired doneness.

-Serve with a whole wheat roll and 1/2 Tbsp of Brumble and Brown butter.

(~401 calories, 40 grams of carbohydrate)

- Chicken Cordon Bleu, winter squash and salad dinner

-Combine 3/4 cup of Italian style whole wheat bread crumbs and ¼ cup of parmesan cheese. Slice a pocket in 4 (6oz) skinless boneless chicken breasts. Stuff each breast with a slice of Swiss cheese and a slice of lean ham. Beat one egg in a shallow dish and dip each stuffed breast in the egg and then dip in bread crumb mixture. Bake chicken at 400 degrees for 15-20 minutes or until chicken is cooked through. Equals 4 (6oz) servings, have one 6oz serving.

-Bake cubed winter squash in 400 degree oven until soft. Mash or leave cubed.

Have one cup with 1 Tbsp of Brumble and Brown butter.

-Have unlimited free salad with a fat free salad dressing.

(~500 calories, 40 grams of carbohydrate)

- Grilled chicken breast, sweet potato fries and broccoli dinner

-Grill 6oz skinless boneless chicken breast brushed with 2 Tbsp of Kikkoman's Teriyaki Baste and Glaze.

-Steam unlimited broccoli and serve with 1 Tbsp of Brumble and Brown margarine and season with salt, pepper and lemon.

-Slice 1 large sweet potato into thin strips, toss with 2 tsp of EVOO and season with salt and pepper. Bake at 400 degrees for 30 minutes or until soft and desired crispiness. Serve with 3 Tbsp of ketchup.

(~400 calories, 55 grams of carbohydrate)

- Whole wheat four cheese ravioli with marinara sauce and salad dinner

- Cook 9oz package of fresh Buitoni whole wheat four cheese ravioli. Makes 2 servings, have one serving with your favorite or homemade marinara sauce (not meat sauce)
- Serve with unlimited free salad with 2 Tbsp of light salad dressing (~600 calories, 80 grams of carbohydrate)

- Whole Wheat 8 inch Boboli pizza crust topped with 1/2cup of your favorite marinara sauce and a 1/2 cup of part skim mozzarella cheese and unlimited veggies. Cook according to pizza crust package. Serve with a free salad topped with 1 tsp of EVOO and unlimited vinegar. (~590 calories, 80 grams of carbohydrate)

- 4.5 ounces (half the package) of Whole wheat four cheese Tortellini with 1 cup of your favorite marinara sauce. Enjoy with a free salad and 2 Tbsp of light dressing. (~615 calories, 75 grams of carbohydrate)

- Grilled Salmon or Tuna, baked potato and asparagus dinner
- Grill 6oz of salmon with 1 tsp of EVOO and lemon
- Bake a russet potato and serve with 1 Tbsp of light sour cream
- Grill asparagus with 1 tsp of EVOO and season with salt and pepper

(~450 calories, 44 grams of carbohydrate)

- 6oz of skinless boneless chicken breast or tenders rubbed with 1 tsp EVOO and Montreal Steak seasoning Grill Mates baked or grilled until cooked through. Serve with steamed broccoli, carrots and snap peas (Green Giant frozen mix) and 1/2 cup of brown rice. (~332 calories, 45 grams of carbohydrate)

Snacks (100-200 calories)

- 6 Triscuit crackers with 1 wedge of light laughing cow cheese (~155calories, 20 grams of Carbohydrate)
- 1 Super Soft pretzel with mustard (~160 calories, 34 grams of Carbohydrate)
- ¾ cup of Low fat Edy's Ice Cream Coffee (or other flavor) (~160 calories, 23 grams of Carbohydrate)
- Whole Wheat baked Pita chips with 2 Tbsp of Hummus (~170 calories, 16grams of Carbohydrate)
- 2 Tbsp of Light Ranch dressing with ½ cup of baby carrots or unlimited cucumbers, peppers, tomatoes etc. (~120 calories, 5 grams of Carbohydrate)
- 2 Tbsp of natural peanut butter with unlimited celery sticks (~200 calories, 6 grams of Carbohydrate)
- Healthy Valley Organic cereal bars strawberry cobbler (130 calories, 27 grams of Carbohydrate)

- 1 Skinny Cow ice cream sandwich low fat vanilla and chocolate (~130 calories, 30 grams of Carbohydrate)
- Stony field vanilla 6oz yogurt (~130calories, 25 grams of Carbohydrate)
- Health Valley Organic multigrain cereal bar (~130 calories, 27grams of carbohydrate)
- 1 100 calorie pack of goldfish (~100 calories, 13 grams of Carbohydrate)
- Healthy Helpings animal crackers (~ 100 calories, 20grams of Carbohydrate)
- 1 Small banana drizzled with 1 Tbsp of Peanut butter (~200 calories, 30 grams of Carbohydrate)
- Chiobanni strawberry yogurt (~140 calories, 20 grams of Carbohydrate)
- 1% fat Cottage Cheese with ¾ cup of sliced peaches (~150 calories, 18 grams of Carbohydrate)

Plate Diagram

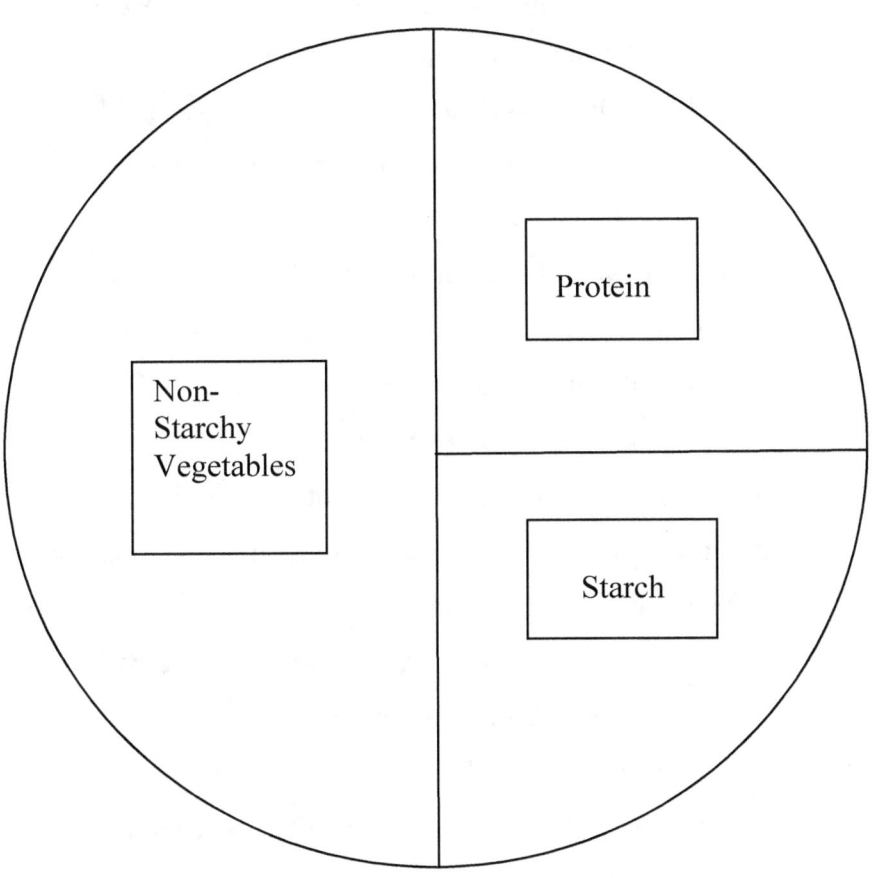

"About the Author"

There have been thousands of books written on weight loss, yet Americans continue to fight obesity. What makes my advice different than what has already been said about the subject is that I am a Registered Dietitian (RD). My diet plan is not a fad diet but instead a way of eating for a healthy life.

Advice on weight loss form an RD is important as it gives you an extra level of assurance that you are learning information from a person who has studied and been certified as an expert in the area of nutrition. To become an RD you must have a minimum of a bachelor's degree in human nutrition from a United States regionally accredited university or college and course work approved by the Commission Accreditation for dietetics education (CADE) of the American Dietetic Association (ADA)". After completing a bachelor's degree an RD must complete an approved 6-12 month dietetic internship. Upon completion of an internship you must pass a national exam administered by the ADA to become and RD. Once you have become and RD you must complete continuing professional education (CPE) credits to keep your RD status current. Registered Dietitians can also call themselves nutritionists but a nutritionist cannot call themselves an RD. You can feel confident that when you are working with Registered Dietitians that they have been through years of training in human nutrition, and must adhere to the strict code of ethics and certification by the ADA and are licensed by the state in which they practice.

Reference List

American Dietetic Association. "Nutrition Fact Sheets."(2008) Available: eatright.org

Beaser, M.D., Richard S., and Amy P. Campbell, R.D, M.S., C.D.E. The Joslin Guide to Diabetes. New York: Simon & Shuster, 2005.

Busch, M.P.H., R.D., F.A.D.A., Felicia. The New Nutrition. New York: John Wiley & Sons, INC., 2000.

Clark, MS, RD, Nancy. Sports Nutrition Guidebook. Illinois: Human Kinetics, 1997.

Groff, James L, Sareen S. Gropper and Sara M. Hunt. Advanced Nutrition and Human Metabolism. New York: West Publishing Company, 1995.

Idaho Plate Method. "The Healthy Diabetes Plate." Available: www.cdc.gov/.../2007/jan/images/06_0050_02. gif

Mahan, Kathleen L. and Sylvia Escott-Stump. Krause's Food, Nutrition, & Diet Therapy. Philadelphia: W.B. Saunders Company,1996.

Mitchell, Mary Kay. Nutrition Across the Lifespan. Philadelphia: W.B. Saunders Company, 1997.

Tortora, Gerard, J. and Sandra Reynolds Grabowski. Principles of Anatomy and Physiology. New York: Harper Collins, 1996.

www.ingramcontent.com/pod-product-compliance
Lightning Source LLC
Chambersburg PA
CBHW060000300526
45794CB00003B/1020